Characterizing E
Agent Orange and Other Herbicides
Used in Vietnam

Interim Findings and Recommendations

Committee on the Assessment of Wartime
Exposure to Herbicides in Vietnam

Board on Health Promotion and Disease Prevention

INSTITUTE OF MEDICINE
OF THE NATIONAL ACADEMIES

THE NATIONAL ACADEMIES PRESS
Washington, D.C.
www.nap.edu

2003

THE NATIONAL ACADEMIES PRESS   500 Fifth Street, N.W.   Washington, DC 20001

NOTICE: The project that is the subject of this report was approved by the Governing Board of the National Research Council, whose members are drawn from the councils of the National Academy of Sciences, the National Academy of Engineering, and the Institute of Medicine. The members of the committee responsible for the report were chosen for their special competences and with regard for appropriate balance.

Support for this project was provided by the US Department of Veterans Affairs. The project was supported by Cooperative Agreement No. V101(93)P-1637 between the National Academy of Sciences and the US Department of Veterans Affairs. The views presented in this report are those of the Institute of Medicine Committee on the Assessment of Wartime Exposure to Herbicides and are not necessarily those of the funding agencies.

International Standard Book Number 0-309-08943-3 (Book)
International Standard Book Number 0-309-51711-7 (PDF)

Additional copies of this report are available from the National Academies Press, 500 Fifth Street, NW, Lockbox 285, Washington, DC 20055; (800) 624-6242 or (202) 334-3313 (in the Washington metropolitan area); Internet, http://www.nap.edu.

For more information about the Institute of Medicine, visit the IOM home page at: **www.iom.edu.**

The serpent has been a symbol of long life, healing, and knowledge among almost all cultures and religions since the beginning of recorded history. The serpent adopted as a logotype by the Institute of Medicine is a relief carving from ancient Greece, now held by the Staatliche Museen in Berlin.

*"Knowing is not enough; we must apply.
Willing is not enough; we must do."*
—Goethe

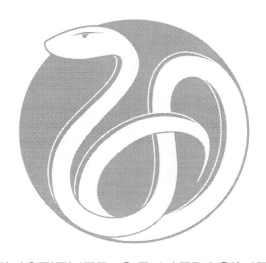

INSTITUTE OF MEDICINE
OF THE NATIONAL ACADEMIES

Shaping the Future for Health

THE NATIONAL ACADEMIES
Advisers to the Nation on Science, Engineering, and Medicine

The **National Academy of Sciences** is a private, nonprofit, self-perpetuating society of distinguished scholars engaged in scientific and engineering research, dedicated to the furtherance of science and technology and to their use for the general welfare. Upon the authority of the charter granted to it by the Congress in 1863, the Academy has a mandate that requires it to advise the federal government on scientific and technical matters. Dr. Bruce M. Alberts is president of the National Academy of Sciences.

The **National Academy of Engineering** was established in 1964, under the charter of the National Academy of Sciences, as a parallel organization of outstanding engineers. It is autonomous in its administration and in the selection of its members, sharing with the National Academy of Sciences the responsibility for advising the federal government. The National Academy of Engineering also sponsors engineering programs aimed at meeting national needs, encourages education and research, and recognizes the superior achievements of engineers. Dr. Wm. A. Wulf is president of the National Academy of Engineering.

The **Institute of Medicine** was established in 1970 by the National Academy of Sciences to secure the services of eminent members of appropriate professions in the examination of policy matters pertaining to the health of the public. The Institute acts under the responsibility given to the National Academy of Sciences by its congressional charter to be an adviser to the federal government and, upon its own initiative, to identify issues of medical care, research, and education. Dr. Harvey V. Fineberg is president of the Institute of Medicine.

The **National Research Council** was organized by the National Academy of Sciences in 1916 to associate the broad community of science and technology with the Academy's purposes of furthering knowledge and advising the federal government. Functioning in accordance with general policies determined by the Academy, the Council has become the principal operating agency of both the National Academy of Sciences and the National Academy of Engineering in providing services to the government, the public, and the scientific and engineering communities. The Council is administered jointly by both Academies and the Institute of Medicine. Dr. Bruce M. Alberts and Dr. Wm. A. Wulf are chair and vice chair, respectively, of the National Research Council.

www.national-academies.org

COMMITTEE ON THE ASSESSMENT OF WARTIME EXPOSURE TO HERBICIDES IN VIETNAM

DAVID G. HOEL* (Chair), Distinguished University Professor, Department of Biometry and Epidemiology, Medical University of South Carolina, Charleston, South Carolina

S. KATHARINE HAMMOND, Professor of Environmental Health Sciences and Director, Industrial Hygiene Program, School of Public Health, University of California, Berkeley, California

LOREN D. KOLLER, Consultant, Environmental Health and Toxicology, Corvallis, Oregon

DANA P. LOOMIS, Associate Professor, Department of Epidemiology, School of Public Health, University of North Carolina at Chapel Hill, North Carolina

THOMAS J. SMITH, Professor of Industrial Hygiene and Director, Industrial Hygiene Program, Department of Environmental Health, Harvard School of Public Health, Boston, Massachusetts

DAVID J. TOLLERUD, Clinical Professor and Associate Director, Institute for Public Health Research, School of Public Health and Information Sciences, University of Louisville, Kentucky

LAUREN ZEISE, Chief, Reproductive and Cancer Hazard Assessment Section, Office of Environmental Health and Hazard Assessment, California Environmental Protection Agency, Berkeley, California

Staff

David A. Butler, Senior Program Officer

Jennifer A. Cohen, Research Associate

James A. Bowers, Project Assistant/Research Assistant (through July 2000)

Anna B. Staton, Research Assistant (through November 2002)

Elizabeth J. Albrigo, Project Assistant

Joe A. Esparza, Project Assistant

Rose Marie Martinez, Director, Board on Health Promotion and Disease Prevention

Kathleen Straton, Acting Director (1997-1999), Board on Health Promotion and Disease Prevention

Rita Gaskins, Administrative Board Assistant

Donna D. Thompson, Administrative Board Assistant (through May 2000

Melissa French, Financial Associate (through June 2002)

Jim Banihashemi, Financial Associate

Norman Grossblatt, Senior Editor

---

*Member, Institute of Medicine

v

Reviewers

This report has been reviewed in draft form by individuals chosen for their diverse perspectives and technical expertise, in accordance with procedures approved by the National Research Council's Report Review Committee. The purpose of this independent review is to provide candid and critical comments that will assist the institution in making its published report as sound as possible and to ensure that the report meets institutional standards of objectivity, evidence, and responsiveness to the study charge. The review comments and draft manuscript remain confidential to protect the integrity of the deliberative process. We wish to thank the following individuals for their review of this report:

Dale B. Hattis, Clark University
Irva Hertz-Picciotto, University of North Carolina at Chapel Hill
Howard M. Kipen, University of Medicine and Dentistry of New Jersey—Robert Wood Johnson Medical School
David F. Utterback, National Institute for Occupational Safety and Health

Although the reviewers listed above have provided many constructive comments and suggestions, they were not asked to endorse the conclusions or recommendations, nor did they see the final draft of the report before its release. The review of this report was overseen by **Jonathan M. Samet**, Johns Hopkins University and **John Ahearne**, Sigma Xi, The Scientific Research Society. Appointed by the National Research Council and Institute of Medicine, they were responsible for making certain that an independent examination of this report was carried out in accordance with institutional procedures and that all review comments were carefully considered. Responsibility for the final content of this report rests entirely with the authoring committee and the institution.

Preface

In response to the concerns voiced by Vietnam veterans and their families, Congress called on the National Academy of Sciences (NAS) to review the scientific evidence on the possible health effects of exposure to Agent Orange and other herbicides (Public Law 102-4, enacted on February 6, 1991). The creation, in 1992, of the NAS, Institute of Medicine (IOM) committee tasked to conduct the review underscored the critical importance of approaching these questions from a nonpartisan scientific standpoint. This study is an outgrowth of that work, focusing on the assessment of wartime exposure to herbicides. The 1994 IOM report *Veterans and Agent Orange* noted that "[e]xposure assessment has been a weak aspect of most epidemiologic studies of Vietnam veterans" (page 18) and recommended that an effort be undertaken to develop models. The US Department of Veterans Affairs asked the IOM to organize the effort, which led to the formation of the Committee on the Assessment of Wartime Exposure to Herbicides.

The committee commends the work of the team of investigators from the Columbia University Mailman School of Public Health (Jeanne Mager Stellman, PhD, Principal Investigator) who carried out the exposure assessment research. Their dogged pursuit of historical records has led to a significant improvement in the quality and completeness of the information on wartime spraying and the individuals who may have been exposed to it. The geographic information system they developed is innovative and serves as an exemplar of how this technology can be exploited in exposure characterization studies. And finally, the spirit of cooperation and collaboration shown by the Columbia University researchers greatly facilitated the Committee's job of oversight and made its task an enjoyable and intellectually engaging one.

David Butler served as the study director for this project. The committee would like to acknowledge the excellent work of IOM staff members Jennifer Cohen, Anna Staton, Elizabeth Albrigo, Joe Esparza, and James Bowers. Thanks are also extended to Melissa French and Jim Banihashemi, who handled the finances for the project; Norman Grossblatt, who edited the manuscript; William McLeod, who conducted database searches; Jennifer Bitticks, who supervised the production of the report; and Rita Gaskins, who provided administrative support to the project.

The committee greatly benefited from the input of scientists, researchers, governmental employees, veterans service organizations, and other interested individuals who generously lent their time and expertise to help give committee members insight on particular issues, provide copies of newly-released research, or answer queries concerning their work or experience. We thank them for their contributions.

David G. Hoel, *Chair*

Contents

INTRODUCTION AND BACKGROUND   1

FOUNDATION FOR FINDINGS   5

OBSERVATIONS REGARDING FUTURE RESEARCH   13

CONCLUSIONS AND RECOMMENDATIONS   14

REFERENCES   15

APPENDIXES

A POWER CALCULATIONS   17

B PUBLIC MEETINGS HELD BY THE COMMITTEE ON THE
   ASSESSMENT OF WARTIME EXPOSURE TO HERBICIDES
   IN VIETNAM   19

C COMMITTEE AND STAFF BIOGRAPHIES   20

Characterizing Exposure of Veterans to Agent Orange and Other Herbicides Used in Vietnam

Interim Findings and Recommendations

INTRODUCTION AND BACKGROUND

From 1962 to 1971, US military forces sprayed more than 19 million gallons of herbicides over Vietnam to strip the thick jungle canopy that helped conceal opposition forces, to destroy crops that enemy forces might depend on, and to clear tall grass and bushes from around the perimeters of US base camps and outlying fire-support bases. Most large-scale spraying operations were conducted from airplanes and helicopters, but herbicides were also sprayed from boats and ground vehicles, and by soldiers wearing back-mounted equipment. After a scientific report concluded that a contaminant of one of the primary chemicals used in the herbicide called Agent Orange could cause birth defects in laboratory animals, US forces suspended use of the herbicide; they subsequently halted all herbicide spraying in Vietnam in 1971.

In response to concerns about the possible health consequences of wartime exposure to herbicides, Congress passed Public Law 102–4, the Agent Orange Act of 1991.[1] The legislation directed the Secretary of Veterans Affairs to request that the National Academy of Sciences conduct a comprehensive review and evaluation of available scientific and medical information regarding the health effects of exposure to Agent Orange, other herbicides used in Vietnam, and their components, in-

---

[1] Codified as 38 USC§1116.

cluding the contaminant 2,3,7,8-tetrachlorodibenzo-*p*-dioxin, informally known as TCDD or dioxin. A committee convened by the Institute of Medicine (IOM) of the National Academies conducted the review and in 1994 published a comprehensive report titled *Veterans and Agent Orange: Health Effects of Herbicides Used in Vietnam* (IOM, 1994).

The committee responsible for the 1994 report encountered a severe lack of information about the exposures of individual Vietnam veterans to herbicides and found that this lack of information had hampered previous attempts to study the effects of exposure to herbicides on the health of Vietnam veterans. That committee felt, however, that it might be possible to develop better methods of determining exposures of individual veterans by drawing on historical reconstructions. The methods might take into account such factors as troop movements, ground and perimeter spraying, herbicide shipments to various military bases, the terrain and foliage typical of the locations sprayed, the military missions of the troops located there, and biochemical techniques for detecting low concentrations of dioxin in the blood. If better models of exposure could be developed and validated, the committee believed, a number of important epidemiologic studies of exposure to herbicides and health outcomes might become possible.

As part of the 1994 report, recommendations were offered concerning the need for additional scientific studies to resolve areas of continuing scientific uncertainty. Three of these recommendations addressed exposure assessment studies of Vietnam veterans (IOM, 1994):

- A nongovernmental organization with appropriate experience in historical exposure reconstruction should be commissioned to develop and test models of herbicide exposure for use in studies of Vietnam veterans.
- The exposure reconstruction models developed according to [the previous recommendation] should be evaluated by an independent, nongovernmental scientific panel established for this purpose.
- If the scientific panel proposed [above] determines that a valid exposure reconstruction model is feasible, the Department of Veterans Affairs and other government agencies should facilitate additional epidemiologic studies of veterans.

In response to that report, the Department of Veterans Affairs (VA) asked IOM to establish a committee to oversee the development and evaluation of models of herbicide exposure for use in studies of Vietnam veterans. That committee would develop and disseminate a request for proposals (RFP) consistent with the recommendations; evaluate the proposals received in response to the RFP and select one or more academic or other nongovernmental research groups to develop the exposure reconstruction model; provide scientific and administrative oversight of the work of the researchers; and evaluate the models developed by the researchers in a report to VA, which would be published for a broader audience.

The Committee on the Assessment of Wartime Exposure to Herbicides in Vietnam was formed in 1996 to accomplish those tasks. Its initial work resulted in the report *Scientific Considerations Regarding a Request for Proposals for Research Characterizing Exposure of Veterans to Agent Orange and Other Herbicides Used in Vietnam* (IOM, 1997). The report—which comprised a statement of work, criteria for selecting researchers, and an appendix providing background information for potential respondents—was released to the public on March 18, 1997. It summarized the RFP's intent as follows (IOM, 1997, p. 3):

> 1. Develop and document a detailed methodology for retrospectively characterizing the exposure of Vietnam veterans to the major herbicides used by the military in Vietnam—2,4-D; 2,4,5-T; cacodylic acid; and picloram—and the trace contaminants TCDD and its congeners. The proposal should address how exposure to this array of chemicals will be evaluated. However, the ability to separately identify or quantify exposures to each of these substances is not necessarily a requirement for a successful proposal. The exposure methodology proposed must be applicable to specific types of epidemiological investigations that could be conducted at a future date under a separate contract or subcontract.
>
> 2. Demonstrate the feasibility and appropriateness of the proposed methodology in sufficient detail to permit the assessment of its potential for use in the conduct of epidemiological studies.

A formal, complete RFP, including the scientific input and contractual requirements, was developed and was issued on June 30, 1997. It was initially sent to individuals and organizations that had requested it or were thought to have an interest in exposure characterization research. Availability of the RFP was publicized on the Web sites of IOM's Board on Health Promotion and Disease Prevention and the Society for Risk Analysis and was posted to relevant e-mail lists. Members of the veteran community and other interested persons were also informed of the RFP through public events held by IOM committees involved in Vietnam veteran health research and through contacts made at meetings and conferences attended by committee members and staff.

Three proposals were submitted by the due date of September 4, 1997. Committee members evaluated the technical and scientific merit of these proposals on the basis of the criteria set forth in the RFP. They concluded unanimously that a proposal submitted by researchers at Columbia University's Mailman School of Public Health (Jeanne Mager

Stellman, PhD, Principal Investigator) merited funding. That conclusion was transmitted to VA on February 24, 1998, and the National Academies initiated a contract with the researchers using funds provided by VA.

The RFP specified that the researchers were to submit scientific progress reports every 6 months over the length of the contract. The progress reports were to include: "a description of the overall progress; descriptions of the specific work accomplished, including problems encountered and corrective actions; pertinent data or other information in sufficient detail to explain significant results achieved and any preliminary conclusions resulting from analysis and scientific evaluation of data accumulated to date; and a description of the work to be accomplished over the following six months" (page 10). Progress reports were presented in public meetings of the committee to disseminate the information to a larger audience and facilitate interaction between the committee and the researchers. The first of these took place in a November 6, 1998, meeting of the committee. Communication was maintained between meetings on a less formal basis.

Discussion between the researchers and the committee played an important role in the project. In addition to being an essential component of the committee's oversight of the contractor's work, it allowed for the work plan to be more easily refined as the project progressed and for the researchers to obtain opinions on alternative means for addressing the challenges and opportunities that presented themselves.

As of January 2003, nine 6-month reviews had been completed. Although the Columbia University effort (as specified in the response to the RFP and modified in consultation with the committee) has not yet been completed, the committee believes that sufficient progress has been made to permit some judgments to be stated.

On the basis of the committee's review of the contractor's 6-month update reports, presentations through month 54, and published and draft papers prepared by the contractor, the committee has reached the following findings:

- The contractor has developed databases of wartime spraying and accidental dispersion of herbicides, of troop locations and movements, and of land features and soil typology.
- The contractor has developed an effective exposure assessment tool to assign a metric—the E4 Exposure Opportunity Index (EOI)—for herbicide exposure that is based on proximity to spraying in space and time and on the amount and agent sprayed.
- The range of calculated EOIs and information gathered to date on troop locations is sufficient to demonstrate the feasibility of future epidemiologic studies. Additional location data for troops not currently in-

cluded in present databases appear to be available at the National Archives for abstraction and use by researchers and other interested parties in future studies.

•   Given current knowledge and available data, the contractor has adequately demonstrated that the draft model is a valid means of assessing wartime herbicide exposure of Vietnam veterans.

On the basis of these findings, the committee concludes that a valid exposure reconstruction model for wartime herbicide exposures of US veterans of Vietnam is feasible. It therefore recommends that the Department of Veterans Affairs and other government agencies facilitate additional epidemiologic studies of veterans by nongovernmental organizations and independent researchers.

The foundation for the findings and the conclusion and recommendation are addressed below. This discussion will make reference to but not reiterate materials published or in preparation for publication by the Columbia University researchers. The committee's 1997 report encouraged the dissemination of scholarly findings resulting from conduct of the research and encouraged dissemination of the findings through publication in peer-reviewed journals. The committee commends the Columbia University researchers for their pursuit of that goal and for their accomplishments. It strongly believes that discussion and publication of the results in scholarly venues strengthens the review process and advances the wide dissemination of the materials.

The committee will continue to oversee the work of the Columbia University researchers. It will produce a second report that will review the completed research effort, transmit the contractor's report and support materials to VA, and offer any additional findings, conclusions, and recommendations that it deems appropriate. The data developed during the research effort will be made available to interested parties without restriction.

FOUNDATION FOR FINDINGS

The contractor has developed databases of wartime spraying and accidental dispersion of herbicides, of troop locations and movements, and of land features and soil typology.

The Columbia University researchers have developed a geographic information system (GIS) into which they have placed an extended and refined database of spray missions and other documented herbicide releases based on the HERBS files discussed in the first National Academy of Sciences report on the effects of herbicide spraying in Vietnam (1974).

This work has led to a substantially expanded inventory of herbicide operations and better information on flight paths of aerial spray missions, number of gallons sprayed (gallonage), and chemical agents. The GIS also includes documented spray mission targets; herbicide storage, transport, and unplanned-dispersal information; military unit identification codes; locations of military units, bases, structures, air fields, and landing zones; movements of combat troops; land features[2]; soil typology; and locations of civilian populations. The development and contents of the GIS are addressed at length in a 2003 *Environmental Health Perspectives* paper published by the Columbia University researchers (Stellman et al., 2003a). As part of this effort, they have expanded and are correcting and validating an archive of previously tracked locations of combat battalions stationed in III Corps Tactical Zone in 1966–1969; this zone was the site of extensive spraying, and the resource may be of great importance in future epidemiologic studies.

The contractor has developed an effective exposure assessment tool to assign a metric—the E4 Exposure Opportunity Index (EOI)—for herbicide exposure that is based on proximity to spraying in time and space and on the amount and agent sprayed.

The databases discussed above form the basis of the computation of the E4 EOI. In brief, this EOI combines the location, gallonage, and herbicide data in the GIS with an environmental-decay factor to generate an estimate of the potential for exposure at a particular location and time. The E4 EOI developed as part of this research has been refined from earlier formulations and now incorporates a more sophisticated methodology and extensive additional data (Stellman et al., 2003a). The Columbia University researchers have made various assumptions regarding the values of variables and how they influence exposure potential, but users may modify the assumptions. A software system that implements the calculation of the E4 EOI is in an advanced stage of development and will be delivered as part of the contractor's final submission.

Figure 1 illustrates the level of detail contained in the GIS.

The range of calculated EOIs and information gathered to date on troop locations is sufficient to demonstrate the feasibility of future epidemiologic studies. Additional location data for troops not currently included in present databases appear to be available at the National Archives for

---

[2] Including coordinates of a variety of features: elevations and land contours, rivers and streams, mountains and highlands, coastal areas and mangrove forests, bays and estuaries, and man-made structures such as roadways and utilities.

abstraction and use by researchers and other interested parties in future studies.

Preliminary experience with the calculation of E4 EOIs suggests that they vary over several orders of magnitude (Stellman et al., 2003a). Figure 2, which illustrates a representative calculation of indices,[3] shows areas of the country where (for the time period shown) there were no known exposures and areas where estimates vary between 10^4 and over 9×10^6. The metric thus appears to have a sufficient range to allow for informative epidemiologic studies of Vietnam veterans.

The Columbia University researchers have developed an approach to classifying military units so that they can be separated by the degree to which their missions required frequent changes in location. That approach has permitted them to develop a database of locations—and changes in location over time—for about 80 percent of all Army troops, most Air Force personnel, and Navy personnel assigned to construction battalions or permanent installations. Their experience indicates that additional location information may well be available in the National Archives and possibly other data repositories (albeit not in an easily accessible form). A how-to manual developed by the Columbia University researchers encapsulates the experience they gained in generating available location information to facilitate future research (Stellman et al., 2002). It must be noted, however, that proper implementation of the model will require effort and expertise on the part of the user.

Given current knowledge and available data, the contractor has adequately demonstrated that the draft model is a valid means of assessing wartime herbicide exposure of Vietnam veterans.

The 1997 IOM report indicated that validation of the exposure assessment approach developed by the contractor was important but that the best method of validation was not obvious and was left to the researchers. The Columbia University researchers have centered their validation efforts on the development of a comprehensive database to which quality control and internal consistency checks have been applied. Those efforts are described in the progress reports submitted to the committee and are addressed in published papers (Stellman et al., 2003a; Stellman et al., 2003b).

The contractor's motivation for taking this approach is that it represents the best means available given the scientific and practical limitations of seemingly more direct validation techniques like biomarker stud-

---

[3] The E4 EOI is quantitative on a ratio scale: an EOI of 1,000 represents twice as much exposure as an EOI of 500.

ies or environmental measurements.[4] Since the methodology they developed bases exposure opportunity scores on the proximity of herbicide releases in space and time, the usefulness of the model depends in part on the precision and completeness of the underlying data.

In brief, their validation work includes

• Comparing and combining disparate versions of the existing herbicide spraying databases to make a single corrected composite record and supplementing it with new mission data from National Archives and other historical records. Those data include leaks, crashes, dumps, and other non-mission-related herbicide releases. Information has also been gathered on bases of operation, airfields, storage depots, and the like to facilitate factoring in of possible undocumented releases.

• Systematically identifying and reviewing possible typographic and reporting errors in the databases and correcting them as appropriate by using primary data and the expert judgment of a consensus panel.

• Creating a database of location histories for military and combat support units by using data from the US Armed Services Center for Research of Unit Records and other documentary sources.

• Combining the more fragmentary records of mobile combat units with expert judgment to develop a way to estimate the location of these troops.

• Evaluating the robustness of the E4 EOI by applying various assumptions to the calculation in a sensitivity analysis. Because the GIS is based on geographic partitions (grids), different breakpoints been have applied to confirm that small shifts in grid parameters do not result in large shifts in estimated exposures.

• Using double-keying and other accepted data-management techniques to minimize the possibility of introducing typographic errors in the entry of new information.

• Developing a quality assurance plan to test all software components of the database and exposure assessment calculation. This plan will be implemented when the model is finalized.

This work provides validation of the inputs to the exposure assessment model. Limited qualitative and quantitative validation information for the model itself is also available. The Columbia University researchers have noted, in presentations to the committee, a correspondence between their database's records of spraying and an independent set of measure-

---

[4] The limitations involved in more-widespread application of such techniques are discussed below.

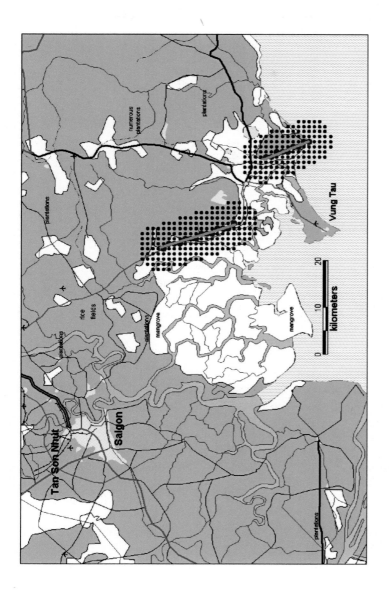

FIGURE 1. Two Agent Orange herbicide missions (numbers 383 and 384, shown as orange lines) flown January 1, 1966, in the Rung Sat Special Zone. Figure shows all grid points whose centers fell within 1 km (large blue dots) and 5 km (small black dots) of the flight paths. +: elevation point; ✈: local airfield.

Source: Contractor presentation made at 42-month update meeting, January 18, 2002, Washington, DC.

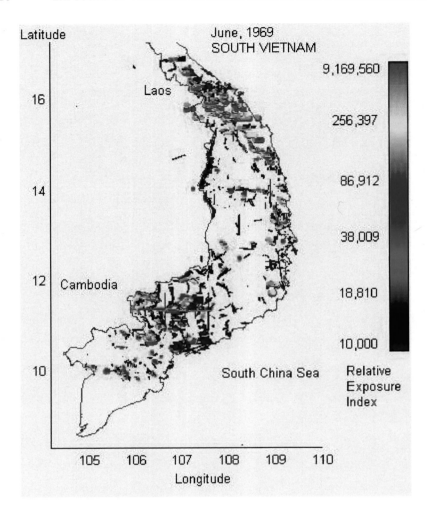

FIGURE 2. Choropleth plot of Vietnam for June 1969 showing exposure potential calculated with the E4 EOI model. Source: adapted from contractor presentation made at 48-month update meeting, July 24, 2002, Washington, DC.

ments made in Vietnam. Dwernychuk et al. (2002) found above-background soil TCDD concentrations in an area of the Aluoi Valley that the Columbia University researchers' database indicates was sprayed with Agent Purple—an early formulation believed to have been highly contaminated with dioxin. Nearby areas that their database indicates were sprayed later with a herbicide formulation thought to have relatively lower dioxin contamination were at background concentrations. The Columbia University researchers also note a 1994 paper (Verger et al.) that found a correlation between dioxin levels in adipose tissue samples of Vietnam residents and an early formulation of their EOI. The paper reported a Pearson correlation coefficient of 0.50 between the log of serum dioxin and the log of the EOI ($p = 0.02$) and a Spearman correlation coefficient of 0.44 for the 22 above-background measurements ($p = 0.04$). When all 27 measurements were factored in, the Pearson correlation coefficient was 0.36 ($p = 0.07$) and the Spearman correlation coefficient 0.32 ($p = 0.10$).

Overall, the committee believes that the Columbia University researchers' work provides an adequate demonstration that the model represents a valid means of assessing wartime herbicide exposure of Vietnam veterans.

The Columbia University researchers have chosen not to conduct a formal analysis of their model with serum dioxin concentrations,[5] other biomarkers, or environmental sampling before submitting it for committee review. The committee supports that decision. While such tests have information value, they are not compulsory for determining whether the model is feasible.

The use of biomarkers to validate an exposure assessment model presents both methodologic and practical challenges. The primary limitation in using present-day serum dioxin concentrations in Vietnam veterans is that too much time has passed since exposure to make them a generally applicable, reliable indicator of exposure. Serum dioxin levels decline over time in the absence of new exposures. For Vietnam veterans, a conservative estimate would predict a decline to less than 10 percent of wartime concentrations.[6] Thus, although the presence of an above-back-

---

[5] Specifically, serum concentrations of 2,3,7,8-tetracholorodibenzo-p-dioxin—the dioxin that contaminated the wartime formulations of some herbicides used in Vietnam. Measurements of other dioxin congeners can provide useful input to epidemiologic studies (Kang et al., 2001), but their presence in serum does not indicate wartime exposure.

[6] Assuming a simple, one-compartment model, a mean TCDD half-life of 7.5 years (Michalek et al., 2002), and an exposure ending on the last day of US wartime involvement in Vietnam (April 20, 1975), a veteran's serum concentration in April 2003 would be 7.5 percent of that when he left the country. If he left 5 years earlier, the figure would be 4.7 percent.

ground concentration in a veteran who has no other known dioxin exposures would strongly suggest wartime exposure, the absence of an above-background concentration does not necessarily indicate that the veteran was not exposed during Vietnam service.

Lack of knowledge about variations in elimination rates poses additional challenges. The pharmacokinetics of dioxin in humans is complex. Current research suggests that the elimination rate depends on several factors, including initial dose, time since exposure, body weight, and sex (IOM, 2003). Therefore, individuals with identical exposures and body burdens during service might not have equal serum concentrations today.

The use of present-day serum dioxin concentrations of Vietnam residents is even more problematic. Vietnam residents experienced different wartime exposures from foreign combatants. Notably, their sole source of food was likely to have been local, and contamination of the food chain is a major source of dioxin exposure (Lorber, 2001). Residents of the south may have also experienced postwar exposure through continued contact with a contaminated environment (Schecter et al., 2001). Dioxin sources other than wartime spraying may be present in various parts of the country, further complicating analysis. Serum measurements taken in Vietnam might provide useful information, but caution would be necessary in evaluating the extent to which this information would validate a model of wartime exposure of veterans.[7] Examination of dioxin concentrations in soil or other ecologic measures might also serve as a check on the accuracy and completeness of spraying records and unintentional releases of some herbicides. However, dioxin fate and transport would need to be accounted for, and the interpretation of current concentrations is not straightforward.

Finally, it must be remembered that not all herbicides used in Vietnam were contaminated with dioxin and that the ones that were had varied and largely uncharacterized levels of contamination. TCDD is a contaminant of 2,4,5-trichlorophenoxyacetic acid (2,4,5-T), a constituent of Agents Orange, Orange II, Purple, Pink, and Green. Agents White[8] and Blue, which together account for about one-third of the gallonage sprayed, were composed of other herbicides.[9] The TCDD concentration in stocks

---

[7] The databases and model created by the Columbia University researchers could be adapted for use in studies of Vietnam residents and may have great utility in this regard.

[8] The National Toxicology Program profile of 2,3,7,8-TCDD noted that it "may be present" in 2,4-D (NTP, 2002), an herbicide used in Agent White. The extent to which dioxin measurements may indicate Agent White exposure is therefore not clear.

[9] Information on herbicide formulations and gallonage sprayed was derived from IOM, 1994 (Table 3-4, p. 89).

of Agent Orange remaining after the conflict ranged from less than 0.05 to almost 50 parts per million (NAS, 1974; Young et al., 1978). Thus, a biomarker study—even one focused on TCDD-contaminated herbicides—would not necessarily yield reliable information on the herbicide exposure of veterans.

Those limitations do not preclude the use of biomarkers or environmental sampling in properly constructed and conducted studies. Indeed, the committee believes that such work is desirable and that the additional information gained from it may lead to refinements of the model. As stated above, however, the committee believes that other available information is sufficient to conclude that the exposure-assessment model is feasible.

OBSERVATIONS REGARDING FUTURE RESEARCH

The committee does not have specific recommendations regarding the type of epidemiologic studies, outcomes, and study populations that should be pursued. It believes that such details are best left to the researchers who are proposing to carry out the work. It can, however, offer some general observations.

Candidate health outcomes for initial study include those for which the committees responsible for the *Veterans and Agent Orange* series of reports have found sufficient evidence of an association with exposure. If the evidence regarding a health outcome is classified as "sufficient", it means that "a positive association has been observed between [herbicide or dioxin exposure] and the outcome in studies in which chance, bias, and confounding can be ruled out with reasonable confidence" (IOM, 1994). There could thus be some reasonable, externally validated expectation that an association might be observed in an epidemiologic study of Vietnam veterans. Appendix A provides the results of sample power calculations to estimate the number of subjects that would be needed to conduct an informative study of one of these health outcomes.

There are several potential candidate populations for such a study. In their 54-month progress report, the Columbia University researchers noted that a study that used a group of veterans that had previously been identified for research or administrative purposes might be initiated relatively easily. Examples include cohorts drawn from the VA Agent Orange Registry, III Corps combat battalions for which location data exist in already-identified National Archives data sources, and cohorts whose locations were documented by the US Armed Services Environmental Support Group[10] as part of previous VA epidemiologic studies. Some military

---

[10] Now the Center for Research of Unit Records.

units maintain detailed histories of their Vietnam experience and active contact with their former members, and they may also present opportunities for epidemiologic research.

The E4 EOI does not measure dose or actual exposure of individuals to herbicides. It is instead a systematic means of classifying potential exposure. Individual dose or exposure measures are the most desirable inputs to epidemiologic studies, but it is often impossible or impractical to obtain them, so researchers routinely assign exposure estimates that are based on indirect or aggregate indexes. That strategy is the norm, for example, in occupational-cohort studies: because individual exposure data are seldom available, workers' exposures are typically assigned from estimates of the average exposure of groups defined by job or work area. Because of individual variations in behavior, biology, and exposure conditions, individuals with identical exposure indexes may have different actual exposures. That is a form of exposure-measurement error. Such errors are typically random with respect to disease status, and in that situation they are likely to cause epidemiologic studies to underestimate the magnitude of any association between exposure and outcome. That potential for bias does not invalidate the use of indexes but instead means that care must be exercised in constructing studies based on such measures and interpreting their results.

It is also important to recognize that an exposure index like the E4 EOI cannot be directly validated or invalidated through an epidemiologic study. Studies based on well-formed hypotheses about outcomes associated with exposure would provide the strongest evidence regarding the validity of exposure estimates. A positive association with an end point strongly believed to be related to herbicides or dioxin in particular would tend to confirm that the E4 EOI measures relevant exposures. However, given the uncertainties inherent in all epidemiologic studies, it is unlikely that any single study could constitute a strong test of validity. Rather, evaluation of the patterns of results from multiple studies would provide guidance as to the performance of the E4 EOI as an indicator of any particular exposure.

CONCLUSIONS AND RECOMMENDATIONS

On the basis of the findings discussed above, the committee concludes that a valid exposure reconstruction model for wartime herbicide exposures of US veterans of Vietnam is feasible.

The committee therefore recommends that the Department of Veterans Affairs and other government agencies facilitate additional epidemiologic studies of veterans by nongovernment organizations and independent researchers. The committee responsible for the 1994 report, in making its recommendations, expressed the opinion that nongovernmental organizations ought to oversee or conduct future studies "to satisfy the public's concern about impartiality and scientific credibility" (IOM, 1994; p. 724). The present committee believes that this approach continues to be the best way to foster both high-quality research and wide acceptance of results.

As noted above, the committee will produce a second, final report that will review the contractor's completed research effort; transmit their report and support materials to the VA; and offer any additional findings, conclusions, and recommendations that it deems appropriate.

REFERENCES

Dwernychuk LW, Cau HD, Hatfield CT, Boivin TG, Hung TM, Dung PT, Thai ND. 2002. Dioxin reservoirs in southern Viet Nam–a legacy of Agent Orange. Chemosphere 47(2):117–137.

IOM (Institute of Medicine). 1994. Veterans and Agent Orange: Health Effects of Herbicides Used in Vietnam. Washington, DC: National Academy Press.

IOM. 1997. Characterizing Exposure of Veterans to Agent Orange and Other Herbicides Used in Vietnam: Scientific Considerations Regarding a Request for Proposals for Research. Washington, DC: National Academy Press.

IOM. 2003. Veterans and Agent Orange: Update 2002. Washington, DC: The National Academies Press.

Kang HK, Dalager NA, Needham LL, Patterson DG, Matanoski GM, Kanchanaraksa S, Lees PSJ. 2001. U.S. Army Chemical Corps Vietnam veterans health study: preliminary results. Chemosphere 43:943–949.

Lorber M. 2001. Indirect exposure assessment at the United States Environmental Protection Agency. Toxicology and Industrial Health. 17(5-10):145–156.

Michalek JE, Pirkle JL, Needham LL, Patterson DG Jr, Caudill SP, Tripathi RC, Mocarelli P. 2002. Pharmacokinetics of 2,3,7,8-tetrachlorodibenzo-*p*-dioxin in Seveso adults and veterans of operation Ranch Hand. Journal of Exposure Analysis and Environmental Epidemiology 12(1):44–53. Corrigendum in 12(2):165.

NAS (National Academy of Sciences). 1974. The Effects of Herbicides in South Vietnam. Part A–Summary and Conclusions. Washington, DC: National Academy of Sciences.

NTP (National Toxicology Program). 2002. 2,3,7,8-tetrachlorodibenzo-*p*-dioxin (TCDD); dioxin, CAS No. 1746-01-6, in 10th Report on Carcinogens. National Toxicology Program, Research Triangle Park, NC, and Bethesda, MD.

Schecter A, Dai LC, Päpke O, Prange J, Constable JD, Matsuda M, Thao VD, Piskac AL. 2001. Recent dioxin contamination from Agent Orange in residents of a southern Vietnam city. Journal of Occupational and Environmental Medicine 43(5):435–443.

Stellman AB, Stellman JM, Stellman SD. 2002. Herbicide Exposure Assessment—Vietnam. User's Manual. Foundation for Worker, Veteran, and Environmental Health, Inc., Brooklyn, NY.

Stellman SD, Stellman JM, Weber T, Tomasallo C, Stellman AB, Christian R. 2003a. A geographic information system for characterizing exposure to Agent Orange and other herbicides in Vietnam. Environmental Health Perspectives 111(3):321–328.

Stellman JM, Stellman SD, Christian R, Weber T, Tomasallo, C. 2003b. The extent and patterns of usage of Agent Orange and other herbicides in Vietnam. Nature 422(6933): 681–687.

Verger P, Cordier S, Thuy LTB, Bard D, Dai LC, Phiet PH, Gonnord M-F, Abenhaim L. 1994. Correlation between dioxin levels in adipose tissue and estimated exposure to Agent Orange in South Vietnamese Residents. Environmental Research 65:226–242.

Young AL, Calcagni JA, Thalken CE, Tremblay JW. 1978. The Toxicology, Environmental Fate, and Human Risk of Herbicide Orange and Its Associated Dioxin. Brooks AFB, Texas: Air Force Occupational and Environmental Health Lab. USAF OEHL-TR-78-92. 262 pp.

Appendix A

Power Calculations

The Columbia University researchers have performed power calculations to estimate the number of subjects that would be needed to conduct an informative study of health outcomes in US veterans of Vietnam. Such calculations comprise many variables, including the incidence rate of the disease being studied, the age of the subjects, the proportion of exposed subjects in the cohort, the statistical confidence levels considered acceptable, and the magnitude of the difference in incidence rates that could be detected.

Illustrative calculations were made for non-Hodgkin's lymphoma (NHL).[1] The sample sizes were estimated on the basis of a 1-tailed chi-square test with alpha = 0.05 and beta = 0.80, an unequal sample size for the exposed and comparison groups (1:4 ratio), and a 587.75/100,000 cumulative NHL incidence in the comparison group. They are given below in terms of the relative risk (RR, also known as the risk ratio) that could be detected.

---

[1] The committees responsible for the *Veterans and Agent Orange* series of reports have found sufficient evidence of an association between exposure to the herbicides used in Vietnam and NHL.

RR	Number exposed	Number comparison	Sample size needed
1.25	23,310	93,240	116,550
1.50	6,356	25,422	31,778
1.75	3,057	12,227	15,283
2.00	1,849	7,395	9,243
2.50	936	3,742	4,677
3.00	590	2,359	2,948
4.00	319	1,273	1,591
5.00	211	842	1,052

All else equal, diseases that are more common than NHL among individuals in the same age bracket as US veterans of Vietnam would require smaller sample sizes to detect the same RR; less common diseases would require larger sample sizes. Using a larger percentage of exposed individuals would also decrease the sample size needed to detect the same RR.

Appendix B
Public Meetings Held by the Committee on the Assessment of Wartime Exposure to Herbicides in Vietnam

MEETING	DATE	LOCATION
6 month update	November 6, 1998	Washington, DC
12 month update	June 1, 1999	Washington, DC
18 month update	December 17, 1999	Washington, DC
24 month update	June 16, 2000	Washington, DC
30 month update	January 12, 2001	Washington, DC
36 month update	July 17, 2001	Washington, DC
42 month update	January 18, 2002	Washington, DC
48 month update	July 24, 2002	Washington, DC
54 month update	January 13, 2003	Irvine, California

Each meeting included presentations of research progress and plans by the contractor and members of the contractor's project staff. All presentations were open to the public.

Appendix C

Committee and Staff Biographies

COMMITTEE ON THE ASSESSMENT OF WARTIME EXPOSURE TO HERBICIDES IN VIETNAM

David G. Hoel, PhD (Chair), is Distinguished University Professor at the Medical University of South Carolina. Dr. Hoel received his AB degree in mathematics and statistics from the University of California, Berkeley and his PhD from the University of North Carolina at Chapel Hill. He is widely published, having been the author or coauthor of more than 150 journal articles and coeditor of several books and journals. Dr. Hoel serves on a variety of national advisory committees and panels, including National Research Council and Institute of Medicine (IOM) committees and the Environmental Protection Agency's Science Advisory Board. He is a Member of the Institute of Medicine, a National Associate of the National Academy of Sciences, and a Fellow of the American Association for the Advancement of Science. Before joining the faculty at the Medical University, Dr. Hoel was director of the division of the National Institute of Environmental Health Sciences with responsibility for the Institute's program in biostatistics, epidemiology, and biochemical and toxicologic risk assessment.

S. Katharine Hammond, PhD, CIH, is Professor of Environmental Health Sciences in the School of Public Health, University of California, Berkeley. Dr. Hammond is a Certified Industrial Hygienist, and her research is focused on exposure characterization. She previously served on the Committee to Review the Health Effects in Vietnam Veterans of Exposure to Herbicides (1994).

Loren D. Koller, DVM, PhD, served in academe for nearly 30 years, the last 16 as Professor in the College of Veterinary Medicine of Oregon State University, Corvallis. For 10 of those years, he served as dean of the college. He operates a business in environmental health and toxicology. Dr. Koller pioneered the discipline now known as immunotoxicology with a research focus also in toxicology, pathology, carcinogenesis, and risk assessment. He served for 6 years as a member of the National Research Council Committee on Toxicology. He also served as a member of the Committee to Review the Health Effects in Vietnam Veterans of Exposure to Herbicides (Third and Fourth Biennial Updates).

Dana Loomis, PhD, is Professor of Epidemiology and Environmental Sciences in the School of Public Health, University of North Carolina at Chapel Hill. His work centers on environmental and occupational epidemiology, and he has published extensively on the characterization of exposure to and risk posed by nonionizing radiation and other physical and chemical agents.

Thomas Smith, PhD, is Professor of Industrial Hygiene in the Department of Environmental Health at the Harvard School of Public Health and Director of the School's industrial hygiene program. Dr. Smith's primary research interest is in the characterization of environmental exposures for studies of health effects. He has developed a toxicokinetic modeling approach for integrating the health effects of toxic substances into epidemiologic studies.

David J. Tollerud, MD, MPH, is Professor and Associate Director of the Institute for Public Health Research, School of Public Health and Information Sciences, University of Louisville, Kentucky. He has extensive clinical training, with specialty-board certifications in internal medicine, pulmonary and critical-care medicine, and occupational medicine. Dr. Tollerud has research expertise in environmental and occupational health, epidemiology, and immunology and consulting experience in occupational and environmental respiratory disease, medical surveillance, and workplace-injury prevention programs. He is an Associate of the IOM and has served as a board member for the Division of Health Promotion and Disease Prevention at IOM since 2001. He has served on a number of Institute of Medicine committees since 1992 and served in leadership roles for the original (1994) and updated (1996) Agent Orange reports.

Lauren Zeise, PhD, is Chief of the Reproductive and Cancer Hazard Assessment Section in the Office of Environmental Health Hazard Assessment of the California Environmental Protection Agency. Dr. Zeise is a toxicologist who has published extensively in exposure assessment and cancer risk assessment.

STAFF

Rose Marie Martinez, ScD, is Director of the Institute of Medicine (IOM) Board on Health Promotion and Disease Prevention. Before joining IOM, she was a senior health researcher at Mathematica Policy Research, where she conducted research on the impact of health-system change on the public-health infrastructure, access to care for vulnerable populations, managed care, and the health-care workforce. Dr. Martinez is a former assistant director for health financing and policy in the US General Accounting Office, where she directed evaluations and policy analysis in national and public health issues. Dr. Martinez received her doctorate from the Johns Hopkins School of Hygiene and Public Health.

Kathleen Stratton, PhD, was Acting Director of the Board on Health Promotion and Disease Prevention of the Institute of Medicine (IOM) from 1997 to 1999. She received a BA in natural sciences from Johns Hopkins University and a PhD from the University of Maryland at Baltimore. After completing a postdoctoral fellowship in the neuropharmacology of phencyclidine compounds at the University of Maryland School of Medicine and in the neurophysiology of second-messenger systems at the Johns Hopkins University School of Medicine, she joined the staff of IOM in 1990. Dr. Stratton has worked on projects in environmental risk assessment, neurotoxicology, the organization of research and services in the Public Health Service, vaccine safety, fetal alcohol syndrome, and vaccine development. She has had primary responsibility for the reports *Adverse Events Associated with Childhood Vaccines: Evidence Bearing on Causality; DPT Vaccine and Chronic Nervous System Dysfunction; Fetal Alcohol Syndrome: Diagnosis, Epidemiology, Prevention, and Treatment;* and *Vaccines for the 21st Century: An Analytic Tool for Prioritization.*

David A. Butler, PhD, is Senior Program Officer in the Institute of Medicine (IOM) Board on Health Promotion and Disease Prevention. He received a BS and a MS in engineering from the University of Rochester and a PhD in public policy analysis from Carnegie-Mellon University. Before joining IOM, Dr. Butler served as an analyst for the US Congress Office of Technology Assessment and was Research Associate in the Department of Environmental Health at the Harvard School of Public Health. He has directed several National Academies studies on environmental-health and risk-assessment topics, including studies that resulted in the reports *Veterans and Agent Orange: Update 1998*; *Veterans and Agent Orange: Update 2000*; *Clearing the Air: Asthma and Indoor Air Exposures*; and Escherichia coli *O157:H7 in Ground Beef: Review of a Risk Assessment*. He is presently directing a study on damp indoor spaces and health—a review of the literature regarding the health consequences of mold and related microbial exposures.

Jennifer A. Cohen is a research associate in the Institute of Medicine (IOM) Board on Health Promotion and Disease Prevention. She received her undergraduate degree in art history from the University of Maryland. She has also been involved with the IOM committees that produced *Clearing the Air: Asthma and Indoor Air Exposures*; Escherichia coli *O157:H7 in Ground Beef*; *Organ Procurement and Transplantation*; *Veterans and Agent Orange: Herbicide/Dioxin Exposure and Type 2 Diabetes*; *Veterans and Agent Orange: Update 2000*; *Veterans and Agent Orange: Herbicide/Dioxin Exposure and Acute Myelogenous Leukemia in the Children of Vietnam Veterans*; and *Veterans and Agent Orange: Update 2002*.

Anna B. Staton, MPA, through October 2002 was a research assistant in the Institute of Medicine (IOM) Board on Health Promotion and Disease Prevention. Ms. Staton joined IOM in December 1999 and worked with the committees that produced *No Time to Lose: Getting More from HIV Prevention*; *Veterans and Agent Orange: Update 2000*; and Escherichia coli *O157:H7 in Ground Beef: Review of a Risk Assessment*. Before joining IOM, she worked at the Baltimore Women's Health Study. Ms. Staton graduated from the University of Maryland Baltimore County with a BA in visual arts (major) and women's studies (minor). She earned her MPA in nonprofit management at the George Washington University School of Business and Public Management.

Elizabeth J. Albrigo is a project assistant in the Institute of Medicine (IOM) Board on Health Promotion and Disease Prevention. She received her undergraduate degree in psychology from the Virginia Polytechnic Institute and State University. She is involved with the IOM Committee on Damp Indoor Spaces and Health. She also helped to facilitate the production of the reports *Veterans and Agent Orange: Update 2002*; *Veterans and Agent Orange: Herbicide/Dioxin Exposure and Acute Myelogenous Leukemia in the Children of Vietnam Veterans*; and Escherichia coli *O157:H7 in Ground Beef: Review of a Risk Assessment*.

Joe A. Esparza is a project assistant in the Institute of Medicine (IOM) Board on Health Promotion and Disease Prevention. He attended Columbia University, where he studied biochemistry. Before joining IOM, he worked with the Board on Agriculture and Natural Resources (BANR) of the National Research Council. While with BANR, he was involved with the committees that produced *Frontiers in Agricultural Research: Food, Health, Environment, and Communities; Air Emissions from Animal Feeding Operations: Current Knowledge, Future Needs;* and *Publicly Funded Agricultural Research and the Changing Structure of US Agriculture.* For the IOM, he assisted on the report *Veterans and Agent Orange: Update 2002.*

James A. Bowers through July 2000 was a project assistant and, later, research assistant in the Institute of Medicine (IOM) Board of Health Promotion and Disease Prevention. He received his undergraduate degree in environmental studies from Binghamton University. He has also been involved with the IOM committees that produced *Characterizing Exposure of Veterans to Agent Orange and Other Herbicides Used in Vietnam; Adequacy of the Comprehensive Clinical Evaluation Program: Nerve Agents; Clearing the Air: Asthma and Indoor Air Exposures;* and *Veterans and Agent Orange: Herbicide/Dioxin Exposure and Type 2 Diabetes.*